The Power of Relevant & Impactful Living

The Power of Relevant & Impactful Living

In Pursuit of Greater Purpose

Dr. T. J. Mdluli

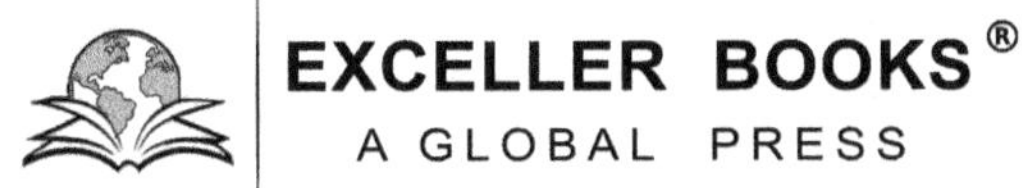

The Power of Relevant and Impactful Living
In Pursuit of Greater Purpose

ISBN: 978-81-19524-40-2

First published in India in 2024 by Exceller Books,
An imprint of GE Group

Address: G1, Dream Apartment, Degree College Road, Belgharia, Kolkata, 700056, India
www.excellerbooks.com

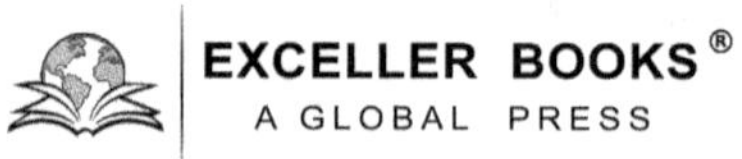

Dedication

To my loving partners, Manasseh group publishers, and Janelle distributors, who have been my constant source of support and inspiration, this journey would be incomplete without you.

Acknowledgement

To my loving wife, Aldiah, who spent countless nights encouraging me and supporting my dream, your unwavering belief in me was my anchor.

My children, your patience and understanding as I spent long hours writing mean the world to me.

To Petros Khoza, whose insightful advice and scholarly guidance shaped the direction of this book, your mentorship has been extremely useful.

Table of Contents

Introduction

Importance and relevance are crucial components of the Christian life. It is our duty as followers of Jesus Christ to live in a way that glorifies God and changes the world for the better. However, it may be all too easy to lose sight of what actually matters most in our fast-paced, distracting environment. This book examines the biblical concepts of influence and relevance and how adopting them might result in a more meaningful and purposeful life. "You are the salt of the earth...you are the light of the world," Jesus tells his disciples in Matthew's gospel (Matthew 5:13-14). We are asked to be a godly influence in our families, churches, and communities, just as salt seasons and preserves. Our words, deeds, and beliefs should direct others toward Christ's healing and hope. Like light, our role in the dark world is to reflect God's love and truth, exposing bad activities and pointing wayward people toward the truth. To be spiritually relevant, one must be a part of the Vine (John 15:5), abiding in Christ via study, prayer, and obedience in order to produce fruit that lasts forever.

Romans 12:2, "And be not conformed to this world: but be ye transformed by the renewing of your mind, that ye may prove what that good, and acceptable, and perfect, will of God is", is an exhortation to believers from the apostle Paul. There is a great temptation to embrace worldly thinking and fit in with the culture. However, God urges us to holy lives that are distinctively Christian and refreshed thoughts that are based on biblical teachings rather than opinion surveys. Our significance stems from boldly adhering to God's perfect will and from transformation led by the Spirit rather than from trying to emulate others.

Being relevant today means being aware of the times, having the discernment to separate fact from fiction, and having the guts to follow God's instructions at all costs. According to Hebrews 10:24, "And let us consider one another to provoke unto love and unto good works" It is our responsibility to hold one another accountable as we encourage one another to grow spiritually and to love and serve one another. Accountability is essential to the church of Christ's continued relevance and edifying influence.

We often judge our lives by materialistic standards such as our social media following, career standing, and material belongings. However, what we accomplished for God's kingdom will be the only thing that matters in the end. "For what shall it profit a man, if he shall gain the whole world, and lose his own soul?" was what Jesus said in Mark 8:36. When we utilize our time, abilities, and resources to further God's mission on earth, sharing the gospel, helping the poor, and modelling Christ by our actions every day, our lives take on eternal meaning.

As Paul states in 1 Corinthians 3:14, "If any man's work abides which he hath built thereupon, he shall receive a reward" is directed at Christians. In the Lord, our work is never in vain. He witnesses our deeds of kindness, tenacity in the face of adversity, and silent prayers of worship. And there is an everlasting reward for those who persevere through the menial and difficult chores. To make an impact on the kingdom, we don't need to be missionaries or pastors. For God, small acts of devotion are important.

Of course, it takes the power of the Holy Spirit to live a meaningful, influential life. In Zechariah 4:6, the Lord of hosts says, "Not by might, nor by power, but by my spirit". Attempting to do God's work alone would only result in failure and exhaustion. The Spirit is our constant source of wisdom, direction, and supernatural empowerment. He will use us to yield fruit that will last an eternity as we surrender to Him daily. All we have to do is follow Him and stay in the Vine.

The following pages examine essential areas in our lives as Christians where we must build impact and relevance. Regardless of our profession, spouses, parents, workers, or churchgoers all have a role to play in the kingdom. In the words of the apostle Peter, "But ye are a chosen generation, a royal priesthood, a holy nation, a peculiar people; that ye should shew forth the praises of him who hath called you out of darkness into his marvellous light." According to 1 Peter 2:9. Let us live as the cherished, specially selected individuals that we are, illuminating the world with our holy light to the glory of God.

Now more than ever, Christians willing to live out their faith with bravery and purpose are needed in a world that is becoming more and more hostile to biblical ideals. "We are not called to shine, we are called to be stars; we are not called to make a difference, we are called to be different," Charles Spurgeon once stated. May the words in this book push and force you to accept genuine significance and long-term influence for God's kingdom. More perfectly seasoned salt and brightly glowing lights are sorely needed in our environment.

Purpose and Overview

In this day and age, there is an urgent need for effective and relevant Christian life. The purpose of this book is to inspire believers to live in a way that glorifies God and expands His kingdom on earth. Hebrews 10:24 reminds us to "consider one another to provoke unto love and unto good works". This book will inspire a passion for living out our faith in ways that matter for eternity through biblical instruction and true anecdotes. Promoting relevance for all ages and contexts is one of the main goals. Though culture changes, human hearts remain the same. The timeless gospel is as relevant today as when Christ walked the earth. By clinging to biblical truth and allowing it to transform our minds, we gain wisdom to engage culture without compromising our witness. As Romans 12:2 states, "And do not be conformed to this world, but be transformed by the renewing of your mind, that you may prove what is that good and acceptable and perfect will of God". God can powerfully use our redeemed lives when we yield ourselves fully.

Outlining the fundamentals for conquering the spirits of mediocrity and inadequacy serves another goal. We must see ourselves the way God sees us, as Spirit-equipped triumphant soldiers, just like Joshua and Caleb did. According to 2 Corinthians 10:4-5, "For the weapons of our warfare are not carnal, but mighty through God to the pulling down of strong holds; Casting down imaginations, and every high thing that exalts itself against the knowledge of God, and bringing into captivity every thought to the obedience of Christ". The only source of our sufficiency is Him. Readers will be encouraged by this book to put their faith in God's strength rather than their own frailty.

This book also seeks to provide believers with the tools they need to overcome spiritual setbacks and apathy. It is possible for believers to gradually lose their spiritual ardour, as Christ cautions in his message to the Laodicean church (Revelation 3:14-22). We are able to be revitalized and returned to our initial love for Christ via repentance, mental regeneration, and dependence on the Spirit. God is the one who gives dead bones new life (Ezekiel 37:1–14). This book will offer helpful strategies for both individual and group spiritual revival.

Ultimately, the central thesis of this book is that, from God's perspective, our earthly labour is never really accomplished. You and I have tasks to complete for the kingdom until He calls us home. "Being confident of this very thing, that he which hath begun a good work in you will perform it until the day of Jesus Christ," Paul wrote in Philippians 1:6. God is constantly shaping, honing, and polishing us so that we might have a bigger influence. As we surrender to His lordship every day, we can have faith that He will accomplish His goals. We just need to hold fast to Him amidst life's ups and downs and have faith that He who started a good job will be faithful to see it through to completion.

An overview such as this offers insight into the topical goal and theme of "The Power of Relevant and Impactful Living." More than ever, Christians who are prepared to make a consistent, lifetime difference for God's kingdom are needed in our world. My hope is that this book will inspire readers to live intentionally for God's glory.

The Power of Relevant and Impactful Living

Living a life of genuine relevance and Christ-centered effect can feel overwhelming in our self-obsessed culture. However, we are called to so much more as followers of Jesus than just aimlessly pursuing unimportant goals in life. In a lost and dying world, our Master urges us to live on a mission, giving of ourselves as salt and light. "See then that ye walk circumspectly, not as fools, but as wise, Redeeming the time, because the days are evil," as Ephesians 5:15–16 warns. There is not much time left to live meaningful lives that will last forever.

Jesus made it clear that we can only produce enduring spiritual fruit by completely living in Him, the Vine (John 15:1-8). Christianity, on the surface, yields little fruit. However, when we develop a close relationship with Christ, we become more relevant and able to benefit others via the power of His Spirit. The rooted existence that provides many with refreshment and nutrition is described in Psalm 1:1–3, which says, Happy is the one who does not follow the unholy advice. However, the Lord's law is what gives him joy, and he thinks about it day and night. And he will resemble a tree planted alongside a river that bears fruit according to the season. A strong internal relationship with Jesus sustains outward relevance and effect.

Of course, it takes more than simply being in God's presence to bear fruit. Even though it hurts, we have to let Him mould and trim us. According to John 15:2, "Every branch in me that beareth not fruit he taketh away: and every branch that beareth fruit, he purgeth it, that it may bring forth more fruit" (KJV). God means trials and tribulations to polish our character, strengthen our faith in

Him, and prepare us for bigger things. As we stick to Christ amid difficulty, we can impact the kingdom.

Living with purpose also entails allocating our time, energy, money, and other resources toward eternal rewards rather than transient pleasures. "Whether therefore ye eat, or drink, or whatsoever ye do, do all to the glory of God," Paul exhorts in 1 Corinthians 10:31 (KJV). Every aspect of life is important for God's purposes. He desires to further His earthly goals with all we have, even insignificant gifts.

Naturally, our talents and good deeds cannot change people's lives. Giving up our role as the Holy Spirit's tools allows for true transformation. Zechariah 4:6 states, "The Lord of hosts saith not by might nor by power, but by my spirit." Self-death is the source of relevance and influence for Christ to live through us. This is the secret to creating a spiritual legacy that endures.

We have the great honour of portraying Jesus daily through our actions in a world that needs salvation and hope. When we walk in obedience to Him, lives are impacted and transformed. May we always submit to His changing work within us so that wherever He sends us, we can be salt and light. In God's eyes, no "small" acts of loyalty exist. Everything accomplished for His honour is of eternal value.

Chapter 1

Living an Impactful Lifestyle

Becoming influential in God's eyes goes beyond the gaudy indicators of success that the public typically praises, such as riches, prestige, and notoriety. Rather, it is based on a close relationship with Jesus Christ marked by steadfast adherence to His teachings and close communion. The eternal alteration of hearts and lives is how this heavenly impact is discerned, not measured by human measures. This life-changing experience is summed up in Romans 12:1, where it is called to live sacrificially. Here, believers are urged to present themselves as living sacrifices wholly dedicated to the service of God. This act of surrender requires laying down every aspect of one's being at the altar of divine purpose, holding nothing back. Through this complete relinquishment of self, the lordship of Christ is established within us, leading to the bearing of fruit that endures for eternity.

Yet, embracing sacrificial living often stands in stark contrast to the inclinations of human nature, which tend to cling to comfort and control. However, by fixing our gaze on the eternal rewards promised by Christ, we find the strength to traverse the narrow path of discipleship. Hebrews 12:2 serves as a poignant reminder of Jesus' unwavering resolve, enduring the cross for the joy set before Him. Similarly, our enduring commitment to the Lord's cause is sustained by the anticipation of His commendation on the final day. The process of becoming vessels of divine impact entails a continuous journey of refinement, wherein God moulds our character into the likeness of His Son. Romans 8:29 elucidates this transformative purpose, affirming God's predestined plan to conform believers to the image of Christ. Through the loving discipline of the Father, our selfish tendencies are gradually replaced by Christlike virtues, enhancing the potency of our testimony before a watching world.

Indeed, the authenticity of our faith finds its most vivid expression through our actions, as emphasized by Jesus' instruction in Matthew 5:16 to let our light shine before others. This luminous testimony serves as a beacon of hope, drawing individuals into the transformative embrace of God's grace. The impact of our witness is magnified when our service to humanity is infused with the love and compassion of Christ, compelling observers to glorify the Father in heaven. However, it is crucial to acknowledge that genuine impact emanates not from human effort but from a posture of abiding in Christ, the True Vine. John 15:1-8 elucidates this symbiotic relationship, underscoring the necessity of remaining connected to Christ to bear fruit that endures. Thus, our endeavours for the kingdom are most fruitful when they flow from a heart surrendered to Christ, attuned to the promptings of the Holy Spirit.

In the midst of our vibrant activism, it is vital to heed the wisdom of Psalm 46:10, which calls us to "be still, and know that I am God." This divine invitation beckons believers to cultivate a spirit of quietude, finding solace and strength in the presence of the Almighty. From this place of intimate communion, our service becomes an outpouring of love rather than a mere religious obligation. The prospect of living an impactful life in partnership with God evokes a profound sense of joy and anticipation. As willing vessels surrendered to the divine will, we become conduits of redemption and restoration, offering hope to the broken and weary souls traversing life's tumultuous journey. May our lives serve as testaments to the transformative power of God's grace as we wholeheartedly devote ourselves to His service, yielding to His guidance and empowerment. Ultimately, our pursuit of impact is not for personal acclaim but for the exaltation of His name and the advancement of His kingdom. In His strength and for His glory, we embrace the privilege of living impactfully.

By embracing the call to live sacrificially, believers embark on a transformative journey of spiritual growth and service to others. This journey, rooted in a deep connection with Jesus Christ, transcends worldly measures of success and instead focuses on the eternal impact of one's actions. As outlined in Romans 12:1, believers are called to present themselves as living sacrifices wholly dedicated to God's service. This act of surrender involves laying down every aspect of one's being at the altar of divine purpose, holding nothing back. Through this complete relinquishment of self, believers invite the lordship of Christ to reign within them, leading to the bearing of fruit that endures for eternity. However, embracing sacrificial living is often challenging, requiring individuals to go against the natural inclination to prioritize comfort and self-preservation. Yet, by fixing our gaze on the eternal rewards promised by Christ, we, the believers, find the strength to walk the narrow path of discipleship. Hebrews 12:2 serves as a powerful reminder of Jesus' unwavering commitment to His mission, enduring the cross for the joy set before Him. Similarly, believers are encouraged to persevere in their devotion to Christ, knowing their labour in the Lord is not in vain.

Becoming vessels of divine impact involves a continuous journey of spiritual formation, wherein God molds believers into the image of His Son. Romans 8:29 elucidates this transformative purpose, affirming God's predestined plan to conform believers to the likeness of Christ. Through the refining work of the Holy Spirit, believers are gradually sanctified, with their selfish tendencies giving way to Christlike virtues. This process not only enhances the potency of believers' testimony but also enables them to reflect the character of Christ to a watching world. Indeed, the authenticity of believers' faith is most vividly demonstrated through their actions, as emphasized by Jesus' instruction in Matthew 5:16 to let their light shine before others. This luminous testimony serves as a beacon of hope, drawing individuals into the transformative embrace of God's grace. The impact of believers' witness is magnified when their service to humanity is motivated by the love and compassion of Christ, prompting observers to glorify the Father in heaven.

However, it is essential to recognize that genuine impact emanates not from human effort but from a posture of abiding in Christ, the True Vine. John 15:1-8 underscores this symbiotic relationship, emphasizing the necessity of remaining connected to Christ to bear fruit that endures. Thus, believers' endeavours for the kingdom are most fruitful when they flow from a heart surrendered to Christ, attuned to the promptings of the Holy Spirit. In the midst of their fervent activism, believers are reminded to heed the wisdom of Psalm 46:10, which calls them to "be still, and know that I am God." This divine invitation beckons believers to cultivate a spirit of quietude, finding solace and strength in the presence of the Almighty. It is from this place of intimate communion that believers' service becomes an outpouring of love rather than a mere religious obligation.

The prospect of living an impactful life in partnership with God evokes a profound sense of joy and anticipation. As willing vessels surrendered to the divine will, believers become conduits of redemption and restoration, offering hope to the broken and weary souls traversing life's tumultuous journey. May their lives serve as testaments to the transformative power of God's grace as they wholeheartedly devote themselves to His service, yielding to His guidance and empowerment. Ultimately, their pursuit of impact is not for personal acclaim but for the exaltation of His name and the advancement of His kingdom. In His strength and for His glory, believers embrace the privilege of living impactfully. By embracing the call to live sacrificially, we should gladly embrace this transformative journey of spiritual growth and service to others. This journey, rooted in a deep connection with Jesus Christ, transcends worldly measures of success and instead focuses on the eternal impact of one's actions. As outlined in Romans 12:1, believers are called to present themselves as living sacrifices wholly dedicated to God's service. This act of surrender involves laying down every aspect of one's being at the altar of divine purpose, holding nothing back. Through this complete relinquishment of self, believers invite the lordship of Christ to reign within them, leading to the bearing of fruit that endures for eternity.

However, embracing sacrificial living is often challenging, as it requires individuals to go against the natural inclination to prioritize comfort and self-preservation. Yet, by fixing their gaze on the eternal rewards promised by Christ, we find the strength to walk the narrow path of discipleship. Hebrews 12:2 serves as a powerful reminder of Jesus' unwavering commitment to His mission, enduring the cross for the joy set before Him. Similarly, believers are encouraged to persevere in their devotion to Christ, knowing that their labour in the Lord is not in vain. The process of becoming vessels of divine impact involves a continuous journey of spiritual formation, wherein God molds believers into the image of His Son. Romans 8:29 elucidates this transformative purpose, affirming God's predestined plan to conform believers to the likeness of Christ. Through the refining work of the Holy Spirit, believers are gradually sanctified, with their selfish tendencies giving way to Christlike virtues. This process not only enhances the potency of believers' testimony but also enables them to reflect the character of Christ to a watching world.

Indeed, as Jesus emphasizes in Matthew 5:16, "Let your light shine before others," the truest testament to a believer's faith is revealed most vividly in their deeds. This brilliant testimony draws people into the life-changing embrace of God's grace like a beacon of hope. When the compassion and love of Christ inspire believers to serve mankind and inspire onlookers to exalt the heavenly Father, the impact of their witness is amplified. But it is crucial to understand that real influence comes from a position of dwelling in Christ, the True Vine, rather than from human effort. This symbiotic relationship is highlighted in John 15:1–8, which emphasizes the need to stay linked to Christ in order to produce fruit that lasts. Therefore, the fruitiest initiatives for the kingdom come from a heart that is yielded to Christ and sensitive to the Holy Spirit's leading.

As Christians engage in intense activism, they should remember the guidance found in Psalm 46:10, which encourages them to "be still, and know that I am God." This divine call encourages believers to develop a calm attitude and find comfort and strength in the Almighty's presence. Believers' service ceases to be only a religious duty and instead becomes an expression of love from this position of close connectedness. There is a great sense of delight and expectation when one considers the possibility of leading a significant life in collaboration with God. Believers become channels of redemption and restoration, bringing hope to the shattered and weary souls navigating life's turbulent journey as willing vessels submitted to the divine will. As they fully commit to serving God and submit to His direction and enablement, may their lives be examples of the transforming power of God's grace. In the end, their goal of making an effect is not to gain recognition for themselves but to elevate His name and further His kingdom. Believers accept the honour of leading influential lives in His might and for His glory.

Understanding the Concept of Impact

Being an impacting person is a goal that is difficult to define since it goes beyond the gaudy measures of popularity and success that the world tends to place a higher priority on. Many people mistakenly believe that having a big impact means controlling enormous ministries, controlling powerful platforms, or enjoying widespread notoriety. Still, true and long-lasting influence frequently springs from the obedient faithfulness displayed in the little, apparently unimportant facets of life. It's like a bricklayer carefully laying one brick on top of the other, piece by piece; building a life that will last forever. This idea is strongly supported by a significant truth that Jesus teaches in Luke 16:10: "He who is faithful in that which is least is faithful also in much..." This passage emphasizes the idea that, even in situations where concrete outcomes may appear elusive, the effect is frequently built through years of endurance in modest acts of service and devotion. God steadily increases people's ability for greater impact as long as they continue to be consistent in carrying out the responsibilities that are allocated to them within their different realms, regardless of how small or seemingly inconsequential they may be. Rather than feeling envious of the apparent grandeur of other people's service spheres, what matters most is the responsible stewardship of the current season.

Even so, human nature still has a tendency to desire instant gratification and tangible rewards for our labours. When real impact seems to be coming at a glacial pace, people are tempted to consider giving up due to feelings of disappointment and disillusionment. But God gently reminds us that His purposes and timing are beyond our limited comprehension. As the poetic passage Isaiah 55:8–9 states, "Because my thoughts are not your thoughts, nor are your ways my ways... My ways are higher than your ways, and my thoughts are higher than your thoughts, just as the skies are higher than the earth." Thus, rather than the observable results that are within God's sovereign control, our influence is ultimately determined by our obedience to His will.

As long as people follow Christ's teachings and submit to the guidance of His Spirit, their lives have an everlasting impact that is well beyond their current grasp. In 1 Corinthians 3:6-7, Paul explains this enigmatic phenomenon by saying, "I have planted, Apollo has watered, but God gave the increase." Thus, God is the one who provides the growth, not the one who plants or waters anything (KJV). In essence, people are supposed to be obedient planters and waterers in God's enormous harvest field, and the outcome is entirely dependent on His favour and His intervention. This awareness does not, however, entail acquiescing in mediocrity or inaction. On the contrary, believers are exhorted in Colossians 3:23 to "do it heartily, as to the Lord, and not unto men." The antidote to complacency lies in the fervent pursuit of excellence in all endeavours, viewing them as acts of worship unto our King rather than mere endeavours to please others. God calls His followers to diligence and wholeheartedness—not in the hope of achieving measurable impact, but as an expression of unwavering fidelity to His will.

Therefore, individuals should take heart even if their ministry or sphere of influence appears modest or insignificant by worldly standards. As aptly stated by Mother Teresa, "We cannot all do great things. but we can do small things with great love." Faithfulness in seemingly inconspicuous tasks has the potential to yield a profound impact over the course of a lifetime spent in communion with Jesus. Consequently, individuals are encouraged to continue laying their bricks, empowered by the indwelling strength of the Holy Spirit. It is imperative to remember that God sees every sacrifice, every act of obedience, and every expression of love offered as worship unto Him. The ultimate reward awaits in His presence.

In a nutshell people shouldn't let short-lived outcomes depress them because real influence isn't always quantifiable in terms of time. Rather, people are called to walk in humility and obedience to God every day, putting their faith in His perfect knowledge and all power. You can be confident that when the right moment comes, the Master will say those precious words, "Well done, good and faithful servant!" Their silent obedience will have had a lasting, incalculable influence.

Let's explore the life of Sarah, a modest woman whose example shows how obedient obedience in the little things can have a profound impact. Sarah was a widow who lived in a small African rural community surrounded by lush vegetation. Sarah had a small amount of resources, but her heart was full of love and compassion for everyone around her. She devoted her days to healing the ill, consoling the bereaved, and lending a sympathetic ear to anyone struggling with life's setbacks. A terrible drought struck the area one fateful day, putting many families on the verge of hunger. Sarah remained resilient while facing hardships.

Rather, she mobilized the neighbourhood, encouraging people to combine their resources and help those in need. Sarah gave food, drink, and clothing to the most in need in the hamlet, showing unshakeable faith in God's provision and providing a ray of hope in the midst of despair. Sarah maintained her commitment in the face of overwhelming difficulty, putting her faith in God's faithfulness to support her efforts. The surrounding villages soon noticed her deeds of generosity and sacrifice and were moved to band together in support of one another. What started out as a modest act of kindness and love quickly developed into a movement of change that impacted the lives of numerous people in the area.

Sarah's legacy persisted for many years after the villages had recovered and the drought had eased. Her unshakable faith and selfless compassion had left a lasting impression on everyone she touched with her goodness. Even though Sarah may never have held a prominent position or led a large ministry, her influence extended well beyond the boundaries of her tiny community and into eternity. Sarah's story is a moving reminder that meaningful life doesn't require big gestures or public attention. Rather, it comes from the obedient humility of people like Sarah, who faithfully manage the opportunities and resources that God has entrusted to them. As we follow in her footsteps, may we, too, leave a loving and compassionate legacy that knows no bounds in space or time, echoing the transformative power of God's grace for future generations.

Embracing Relevancy in All Generations

It is difficult to stay spiritually relevant in a culture that is always evolving. Biblical truth can appear outdated or irrelevant as new technology, beliefs, and worldviews develop with every generation. However, God calls us to share the timeless message in relevant ways with each new generation. But how can we uphold the infallible principles of Scripture while embracing relevance across the generations?

Above all, we must base our relevance on God's everlasting Word rather than just following fads in society. As Isaiah 40:8 proclaims, "The grass withereth, the flower fadeth: but the word of our God shall stand forever." Despite the ever-shifting sands of culture, God's truth remains steadfast and unchanging, serving as a fixed reference point for navigating through shifting times. Our calling is to faithfully proclaim and live out His unchanging gospel, even when it appears to be out of step with prevailing cultural norms. However, while the message remains constant, the methods of communication and application must be prayerfully discerned to resonate with each generation. As the apostle Paul articulated in 1 Corinthians 9:22-23, "I am made all things to all men, that I might by all means save some. And this I do for the gospel's sake..." Effectively presenting the gospel requires understanding our audience and speaking their language while steadfastly maintaining the integrity of the message itself.

Reaching younger generations for Christ necessitates intentionally building meaningful relationships with them. Jesus' example underscores the importance of demonstrating genuine care and empathy, for people do not typically heed what we say until they know that we genuinely care about them. To effectively engage with younger generations, we must take the time to understand their hopes, struggles, and beliefs, as rushing to impart truth without first establishing rapport leads to the construction of barriers rather than the building of bridges. Patience is also a vital virtue when engaging cross-generationally. In 1 Timothy 4:12, Paul admonishes Timothy, saying, "Let no man despise thy youth; but be thou an example of the believers, in word, in conversation, in charity, in spirit, in faith, in purity." Young believers possess valuable insights and perspectives that can enrich the faith community if seasoned saints are willing to listen, gently mentor, and appreciate their contributions. Similarly, older Christians must be willing to graciously receive wisdom from younger ones, recognizing that God can speak through individuals of all ages.

Nevertheless, it is important to recognize that cultural relevance has its limits. In Romans 12:2, Paul cautions against being "conformed to this world" but rather encourages believers to be transformed by renewing their minds. While engaging with culture and adapting our communication methods is essential, we must guard against compromising our beliefs and witness in the pursuit of relevance. Ultimately, our allegiance is first and foremost to our King, Jesus Christ, and our actual significance comes from the Holy Spirit working through surrendered lives. In the final analysis, Christ Himself, the Living Word, ensures that our message remains relevant and life-changing for all generations. As Jesus Himself declared in Luke 21:33, "Heaven and earth shall pass away: but my words shall not pass away." Our primary task is not to reinvent the gospel or cater to cultural whims but to centre our lives wholly on Christ—abiding in Him, listening to Him, and proclaiming Him. As we exalt Jesus alone, His Spirit draws hungry souls across every generation who long to know Him.

Embracing relevancy in ministry requires much prayer, patience, and love. Yet, God equips us for this noble task as we wholly rely on Him. By abiding in His enduring Word, applying it with discernment, building meaningful relationships, and focusing solely on Christ, we can bear fruit that impacts generations to come until He returns. Our relevance truly rests in Him alone.

Let me share the story of Jonathan, a young man who navigated the complexities of cultural relevance while remaining anchored in the timeless truths of Scripture. Jonathan grew up in a bustling city, surrounded by diverse cultural influences and societal pressures. As he matured in his faith, Jonathan felt a deep burden to reach his peers with the gospel message, yet he grappled with how to communicate it effectively in a rapidly changing cultural landscape. Jonathan began by immersing himself in God's Word, seeking to understand its timeless principles and how they could be applied to the realities of contemporary life. He spent hours in prayer, asking God for wisdom and discernment in navigating the complexities of cultural relevance. Jonathan also sought the guidance of older, more seasoned believers who could offer insights gleaned from their own experiences.

Armed with a solid foundation in Scripture and the wisdom of mentors, Jonathan set out to engage with his peers in meaningful ways. He volunteered at a local youth centre, where he built relationships with at-risk teens and provided a listening ear to their struggles and concerns. Jonathan also used social media platforms to share snippets of biblical truth in a manner that resonated with his generation, always mindful of maintaining the integrity of the gospel message. Despite facing occasional pushback and scepticism from his peers, Jonathan remained steadfast in his commitment to Christ and His Word. He refused to compromise his beliefs or water down the gospel in pursuit of cultural relevance, trusting instead in the power of the Holy Spirit to convict hearts and transform lives. Over time, Jonathan's genuine love for others and unwavering faith in Christ began to bear fruit, as several of his friends and acquaintances came to faith in Jesus Christ.

Jonathan's story serves as a powerful reminder that remaining spiritually relevant in an ever-changing culture requires a firm foundation in God's Word and a willingness to engage with others in meaningful ways. By abiding in Christ and faithfully proclaiming His truth, believers can navigate the complexities of cultural relevance while remaining anchored in the timeless truths of Scripture.

Chapter 2

Overcoming the Spirit of Inadequacy & Mediocrity

Fighting emotions of inadequacy, inferiority, or being "less than" is a common problem on the spiritual path. It's in a world where performance metrics and social expectations rule the day; it's simple to fall into the trap of judging our value by things outside of ourselves, like abilities, accomplishments, or other people's approval. Instead, we should ground ourselves on the unwavering reality of God's perfect love. Scripture, however, invites us to view ourselves through the prism of divine truth, reassuring us of our intrinsic value and function as God's cherished children. The words of 2 Timothy 1:7 resonate deeply within the hearts of believers, offering solace and assurance: "For God hath not given us the spirit of fear; but of power, and love, and a sound mind." These words serve as a beacon of hope, reminding us that our identity is not contingent upon worldly accolades or achievements but is firmly rooted in being cherished children of the Creator. God equips us with the power, purpose, and mental clarity needed to walk confidently in our divine calling through His Spirit. In His eyes, we are not inadequate or mediocre; we are fearfully and wonderfully made, destined for greatness in His Kingdom.

Yet, despite the assurances of Scripture, the temptation to compare ourselves unfavourably to others often lingers. 1 Corinthians 12:14-18 offers a poignant reminder of the equal worth and significance of every member within the body of Christ. Regardless of their perceived talents or roles, each individual contributes uniquely to the body's overall functioning. Just as the hand cannot say to the foot, "I do not need you," so too does God design interdependence among His children. Our place within the body is vital and complete, and the talents of others do not diminish the gifts and calling that God has bestowed upon us.

Moreover, the presence of individuals we perceive as more accomplished or talented can often exacerbate feelings of inadequacy or mediocrity. Yet, God intentionally places us in such situations to remind us that true fruitfulness stems from abiding in Him rather than striving in our own strength (John 15:5). As 2 Corinthians 12:9 reassures us, "My grace is sufficient for thee: for my strength is made perfect in weakness." Our sufficiency and adequacy come not from our own abilities but from Christ alone.

To fully embrace our identity and worth as children of God, we must actively renew our minds with the truth of God's Word rather than conforming to the messages of the surrounding culture (Romans 12:2). Immersing ourselves in Scripture allows us to perceive ourselves as God sees us and instills within us the confidence to offer our imperfect gifts and talents back to Him. As we understand who we are in Christ, we gain the courage to step out boldly for the sake of His Kingdom, knowing that His Spirit within us equips us for every good work (2 Timothy 1:6-7). God calls us to serve Him with boldness and confidence rather than allowing feelings of inadequacy or fear to paralyse us. Psalm 139:14 celebrates the intricacies of God's creation, declaring, "I will praise thee; for I am fearfully and wonderfully made: marvellous are thy works; and that my soul knoweth right well." Each of us is uniquely designed by God, with specific personalities, stories, and spiritual gifts, and we have a distinct kingdom purpose unlike any other.

To illustrate this truth, let me share the story of Sarah, a young woman who wrestled with feelings of inadequacy and inferiority in her faith journey. Despite her deep love for God and earnest desire to serve Him, Sarah often found herself plagued by self-doubt and comparison as she witnessed the accomplishments and talents of others in her church community. Whether it was leading worship, teaching Sunday school, or participating in outreach activities, Sarah couldn't help but feel like she didn't measure up to her peers' perceived success standards. One day, while attending a church event, Sarah had a chance encounter with an elderly woman named Mrs. Jenkins. Despite her advanced age and frail appearance, Mrs Jenkins exuded a sense of peace and contentment that captivated Sarah's attention. Over a cup of tea, Sarah poured out her heart to Mrs Jenkins, confessing her struggles with feelings of inadequacy and self-doubt in her faith journey.

To Sarah's surprise, Mrs. Jenkins listened intently, nodding sympathetically as she shared her own experiences of wrestling with similar feelings in her youth. Yet, despite her struggles, Mrs. Jenkins recounted how God had used her in remarkable ways over the years, not because of her talents or achievements, but simply because of her willingness to surrender to His leading and trust in His faithfulness. As Sarah listened to Mrs Jenkins' stories of faith and perseverance, she realised that her worth and identity were not defined by her accomplishments or the opinions of others but by her relationship with her Heavenly Father.

Inspired by Mrs. Jenkins' example, Sarah embraced her unique calling and trusted God's sufficiency to work through her weaknesses.

In the following weeks and months, Sarah stepped out in faith, serving God with renewed confidence and boldness. Whether it was leading a small group, volunteering in the community, or simply offering a listening ear to those in need, Sarah discovered the joy and fulfilment that comes from surrendering to God's plan for her life. And though she still faced moments of doubt and insecurity, Sarah took comfort in knowing that her worth and purpose were secure in Christ alone. Therefore, embracing our worth and purpose as beloved children of God is filled with challenges and triumphs. Yet, as we anchor ourselves in the unshakable truth of God's Word and trust in His faithfulness, we can find the courage to overcome feelings of inadequacy and step boldly into the unique calling He has placed on our lives. And like Sarah, may we find inspiration and encouragement in the stories of those who have gone before us, reminding us that our worth and identity are found in Christ alone.

Identifying and Addressing Inadequacy

It's understandable to feel inadequate at times in this fast-paced, high-achieving world. Social media profiles and carefully curated images feed the lie that everyone else is thriving except us. In reality, we all have weaknesses, flaws, and limitations - yet God specialises in using inadequate vessels! The key is humbly acknowledging our insufficiencies and allowing Him to empower us in those areas. As Romans 3:23 reminds us, "All have sinned and come short of the glory of God." We are all incomplete works in progress on this side of eternity. The healthiest approach is not denying our flaws but inviting God's light to expose them so His strength can shine through. As Isaiah 64:8 states, "We are the clay, thou our potter." Yielding to Potter's shaping and moulding allows beauty to emerge.

Of course, acknowledging inadequacy first requires noticing it. We often live on autopilot, not assessing our lives against God's truth. 2 Corinthians 13:5 challenges believers, "Examine yourselves, whether ye be in the faith; prove your own selves." Taking time for prayerful self-examination helps reveal areas where we fall short of God's best - impatience, discontentment, selfishness, and more. Once inadequacies surface, we can take action through God's power. James 1:22 instructs, "But be ye doers of the word, and not hearers only." Simply feeling guilty changes nothing. True transformation happens by applying biblical truth to our specific weaknesses. Replace lies with God's promises. Study Jesus' example. Seek accountability and counselling. Small steps of obedience make a difference over time.

Of course, addressing inadequacy requires grace towards ourselves. The Father is far more patient with our flaws than we are! As Psalm 103:14 says, "For he knoweth our frame; he remembereth that we are dust." And Isaiah 42:3 promises, "A bruised reed shall he not break, and the smoking flax shall he not quench." God handles us gently, not crushing damaged reeds or extinguishing flickering faith. We can extend the same grace toward ourselves. As we take steps to grow, we must remember that inadequacy has a purpose - keeping us dependent on the True Vine. Jesus said in John 15:5, "I am the vine, ye are the branches: He that abideth in me, and I in him, the same bringeth forth much fruit: for without me ye can do nothing." Our flaws provide opportunities for Christ's strength to shine if we rely fully on Him.

While inadequacies may be part of our earthly journey, they need not paralyse us from God's purposes. 2 Corinthians 12:9 promises, "My grace is sufficient for thee: for my strength is made perfect in weakness." In humility and trust, we can step out to live boldly. For when we are weak, then He is strong. Rather than being discouraged by flaws, see them as reminders to cling to the Vine. He loves using imperfect vessels who lean wholly on Him. Our inadequacies provide openings for His light to shine through the cracks. What matters most is walking in intimacy with Jesus, the flawless One. He completes all that is lacking in us.

Principles for Rising above Mediocrity

God created each of us with unique talents and a high calling, not content with halfway obedience or mediocre living. Though mediocrity tries lulling us into complacency, we serve the King of kings, called to live boldly on a mission for His glory. What principles help us rise above spiritual mediocrity?

My first recommendation is to pursue growth and learning. Proverbs 18:15 urges us to keep expanding our knowledge and abilities: "The heart of the prudent getteth knowledge; and the ear of the wise seeketh knowledge." Mediocrity thrives in stagnancy, but passionate learners avoid spiritual sluggishness. Read challenging books. Listen to inspiring teachings. Seek out mentors. Ask questions. Remain teachable and hungry, no matter your age. Keep adding fuel to your faith.

Also, adopt an attitude of excellence. God commands his people in Deuteronomy 6:18 to "do that which is right and good in the sight of the Lord." Our work belongs to Him; are we giving Him our leftovers or the very best? Colossians 3:23 challenges, "And whatsoever ye do, do it heartily, as to the Lord, and not unto men." Pursuing excellence shows reverence and lifts our work from drudgery to worship.

Next to that, refuse comparison. Seeing gifts and fruit in others can lead to either pride or jealousy, rooting us in mediocrity. Paul charges in Galatians 6:4, "But let every man prove his own work, and then shall he have to rejoice in himself alone, and not in another." Keep your eyes on your own race, the calling God specifically gave you. Run with endurance; His affirmation is all we need.

Additionally, get out of ruts and comfort zones. The temptation toward complacency is real. But Revelation 3:2 warns the lukewarm that Jesus will spit them from His mouth! He wants on-fire devotion, not half-heartedness. Regularly ask God to revitalise areas of your life that have grown stale. Listen for His nudges toward new ventures. Be willing to step into unknowns with Him.

Don't forget this: We serve the King of kings. Jesus urges His servants in Luke 12:48, "For unto whomsoever much is given, of him shall be much required." We are not our own but bought at an infinite price by the Lord of Lords. He deserves the full offering of our gifts and talents, not leftovers. Bring Him your very best each day.

Of course, relying on the empowering Holy Spirit is the ultimate key to rising above mediocrity. Zechariah 4:6 promises, "Not by might nor by power, but by my Spirit, says the Lord Almighty." We remain spiritually vibrant not by trying harder in our inadequate strength but by continually drawing near to Jesus. Abide in the True Vine, and His life flows through you. Beloved child of the Most High, you were created for more than average! Shake off mediocrity's shackles by pursuing growth, excellence, and intimacy with Christ daily. Fix your eyes upon Jesus, the Author and Perfecter of faith. His Spirit in you enables you to transcend mediocrity and live boldly for His glory. You have a noble calling worthy of your best. Go in His power!

Chapter 3
Maintaining Spiritual Momentum - Lessons from Joshua & Caleb

In a culture of spiritual sluggishness, how can we maintain passion and momentum in following Jesus? The examples of Joshua and Caleb in the Old Testament provide inspiring models of persevering faith and zeal. Though facing trials in the wilderness, they never wavered from wholehearted devotion to God. What timeless principles can we learn from these spiritual champions?

Joshua and Caleb possessed a bold vision of God's promises. When 10 of the 12 spies cowardly claimed the giants in Canaan were too strong, Joshua and Caleb saw through the eyes of faith. Numbers 14:7-9 records Caleb quieting the Israelites, declaring, "The land...is an exceedingly good land. If the Lord delight in us, then he will bring us into this land and give it to us." Despite overwhelming odds, they relied on God's covenant promises. Do we cling to God's Word when circumstances look bleak?

They rejected a negative mentality. While the other spies spread fear, Joshua and Caleb urged the people to trust the Lord in Numbers 14:9, saying, "Rebel not ye against the Lord, neither fear ye the people of the land...the Lord is with us." They refused to be swayed by naysayers and grumblers, anchoring their minds to God's truth. Negativity is toxic to spiritual passion. We must guard our minds against faith-sapping thoughts.

The next was they wholly followed the Lord. Of that wilderness generation, only Joshua and Caleb later entered the Promised Land because "they followed the Lord fully" (Numbers 32:11-12). Half-heartedness with God leads to spiritual lethargy. These two men modelled radical, unwavering obedience. Their passion came from forsaking all to follow God. We must cling to Him alone, not divided loyalties that erode zeal.

They trusted God to defeat giants. Though facing powerful enemies, Joshua and Caleb believed God could overcome them. After 45 years, Caleb, then 85, boldly requested the stronghold of Hebron, saying in Joshua 14:12, "If so be the Lord will be with me, then I shall be able to drive them out." His confidence rested in the Lord's power, not his strength. He lived boldly because his faith was in God. We must believe He will defeat our giants.

After which, they patiently endured testing. The wilderness years surely challenged these men's stamina and hope. But they persevered in faith to gain promised victory. We must embrace seasons of waiting and difficulty rather than resenting them. James 1:3-4 reminds us, "The trying of your faith worketh patience...that ye may be perfect and entire, wanting nothing." Trials strengthen spiritual muscles. Joshua and Caleb show us passionate commitment despite long tests.

Like Joshua and Caleb, may we tenaciously embrace God's promises, reject negativity, pursue undivided obedience, rely on God's power, and patiently endure trials. The world desperately needs more champions like these courageous men to live wholeheartedly for the Lord. God seeks those who will stand in the gap to lead others to His best. As Psalm 37:23-24 encourages, when walking with God, "The steps of a good man are ordered by the Lord: and he delighteth in his way. Though he falls, he shall not be utterly cast down: for the Lord upholds him with his hand." When we commit our way to the Lord, He sustains spiritual momentum even through failures and valleys. By His grace, may we "press toward the mark for the prize of God's high calling in Christ Jesus" (Philippians 3:14). Let us run our race with persevering passion like Joshua and Caleb. With the Spirit's help, we will finish strong.

Examining the Lives of Joshua and Caleb

In the biblical account of Israel's wilderness wanderings, two men stand out for their extraordinary faith and courage: Joshua and Caleb. While the unbelieving generation they belonged to perished in the desert, Joshua and Caleb fully followed the Lord and received the promise. What set these giants of the faith apart, and what lessons can we glean from their exemplary lives?

First, Scripture testifies that Joshua and Caleb wholly followed the Lord with undivided hearts. Numbers 32:12 states God's assessment that they "wholly followed the Lord." No other wilderness generation members earned this distinction. Joshua and Caleb's passion sprang from forsaking all competing loyalties to cling to the Lord alone. We see this modelled in Joshua 24:15, when Joshua boldly declares, "As for me and my house, we will serve the Lord." Single-minded devotion to God fueled their faith.

Secondly, they embraced God's promises with tenacious belief despite impossible circumstances. When ten faithless spies gave a bad report on Canaan, only Caleb and Joshua insisted in Numbers 13:30 that "we are well able to overcome it." They anchored their hope to the certainty of God's covenant promises, not earthly limitations. This resilient faith enabled them to stand strong when all others fell away. Their trust was in the Almighty's faithfulness, not human strength or Probability. In addition, they wholly relied on the Lord's power to conquer giants. After 45 years, 85-year-old Caleb boldly approached Joshua in Joshua 14:10-12 requesting Hebron, saying, "The Lord will be with me, and I shall drive them out." At an age of feebleness, Caleb's confidence rested solely in the Lord's enablement to overcome formidable enemies. He and Joshua understood victory would come only through His mighty hand, not their own might.

Furthermore, Joshua and Caleb refused to be swayed by negative voices. As the ten faithless spies spread fear through the congregation, these two men tore their clothes and exhorted the people in Numbers 14:9 to not rebel, for the Lord would lead them to victory. Though standing alone, they refused to echo the voice of unbelief. Their righteous courage stemmed from filtering out naysayers and fixing their eyes on Almighty God. They modelled perseverance through long seasons of testing. After their bold stand, Joshua and Caleb wandered for 40 more years with the faithless generation. Certainly, fatigue and discouragement assaulted their hope at times. But they endured the refining fire and emerged as champions of faith. Their passion was undimmed by delays because they awaited God's perfect timing. They exemplify enduring hope.

The lives of Joshua and Caleb remind us to ground our passion and courage in God's proven faithfulness, not fleeting emotions. When we wholly follow Christ with undivided hearts, we become unshakable "living stones" fueled by his spirit. Jesus declared in John 14:21, "He who has My commandments and keeps them, it is he who loves Me. And he who loves Me will be loved by My Father, and I will love him and manifest Myself to him." May we passionately obey our Lord with persevering faith until the end, like Joshua and Caleb.

Practical Steps for Sustaining Spiritual Momentum

Maintaining passion and zeal in following Jesus can feel challenging in our fast-paced, distracting world. When spiritual momentum ebbs, it is easy to coast in complacency rather than cultivating an intimate walk with Christ. What practical steps can help us retain a fiery faith over the long haul? Immersing ourselves in Scripture sustains spiritual vibrancy. Jesus prayed to the Father in John 17:17, "Sanctify them through thy truth: thy word is truth." As we engage God's Word, it transforms our minds and renews our passion for obedience. Just as we feed our bodies physical food, we must feast on the Bread of Life daily for nourishment. Setting aside time to study, memorize and meditate on the Bible fuels spiritual life.

Pursuing prayer preserves the fervency of spirit. 1 Thessalonians 5:17 simply commands, "Pray without ceasing." Bringing all aspects of life—struggles, temptations, decisions, dreams—to the Lord in prayer reminds us of our utter dependence on Him. Just as any relationship decays without communication, our connection to God erodes without consistent prayer. Pouring out our hearts to the Father fans the flames of spiritual zeal.

Also, gathering regularly with fellow believers stimulates passion for God's Kingdom. In Hebrews 10:24-25, the author warns against neglecting to meet together but encourage each other. The communal nature of our faith was designed to stir up mutual love and good works. Accountability, worship and Word-centered teaching in the Christian community helps protect against stagnancy or backsliding. In addition, serving others combats complacency by directing focus outward. Paul exhorts in Galatians 5:13, "By love serve one another." Using our gifts to meet practical needs with agape love keeps us from idleness that breeds apathy. Engaging in Kingdom work alongside fellow saints unifies and energizes the body of Christ.

Carefully monitoring personal influences aids consistency. Paul instructs in 1 Corinthians 15:33, "Do not be deceived: Bad company ruins good morals." Those we open our hearts to shape our thinking, passions and discipline. Avoiding relationships that quench spiritual zeal safeguards momentum. Wise mentors spur us toward Christlikeness. Of course, sustaining lifelong passion, above all, requires abiding in Christ. Jesus said in John 15:4-5, "Abide in me and I in you. As the branch cannot bear fruit by itself unless it abides in the vine, neither can you unless you abide in me." No amount of diligence avails without drawing life from the Vine. Only through clinging wholly to Jesus will our inner fire continue burning bright for the long haul. May we surrender daily to His Spirit's leading? By God's grace, applying these practical steps positions us to finish the race with endurance and relentless passion. With faces set like flint, may we tenaciously pursue intimate fellowship with Christ every moment until we see His face. Fan the flame within! Our Savior is worthy of a lifetime of wholehearted devotion.

Chapter 4

Bouncing Back from Adversity

Life often deals unexpected blows through hardship, tragedy, illness, relational ruptures, and dreams deferred. When adversity strikes, our first reactions are typically shock, anger, or despair. However, the true test of character is whether we get stuck in defeatism or courageously bounce back. As believers, how can we demonstrate resilience and hope in the midst of trials? We must anchor our perspective to God's sovereign plan, not life's interruptions. The Apostle Paul modelled this mindset after his arrest in Jerusalem, declaring in Acts 20:24, "But I do not account my life of any value nor as precious to myself, if only I may finish my course and the ministry that I received from the Lord Jesus." Despite adversity, Paul's eyes remained fixed on fulfilling his God-given mission. Remembering our lives belong to God helps us view setbacks on a canvas bigger than one moment.

Call to remembrance of God's past faithfulness. The Psalmist frequently rehearsed the Lord's goodness to encourage his soul during hardship. "Lord, you alone are my portion...The lines have fallen for me in pleasant places; indeed, I have a beautiful inheritance" (Psalm 16:5-6). Thanking God for previous graces strengthens courage that He will continue to carry us through present trials. His steadfast love is our life raft amid the storm. Also, learn to lean into the biblical community for support and perspective. Attempting to soldier through adversity alone often proves overwhelming. Ecclesiastes 4:9-10 reminds us, "Two are better than one...For if they fall, one will lift up his fellow." God designed His body to uphold the weary and wounded. Seeking counsel, prayer, and encouragement from trusted fellow believers provides a reflective mirror of Christ's comfort to help us bounce back.

Persevering faith trusts God's perfect timing over our desire for control. Joseph demonstrated radical trust in God's promise as he endured unjust imprisonment, holding to hope for thirteen long years (Genesis 37-50). Likewise, as we walk through seasons of hardship or waiting, we can rest in the knowledge that God's delay is never God's denial. His timing is perfect, even when we don't understand. Look for evidence of God's redemptive hand already at work in the trial. Paul reassures believers in Romans 8:28, "For those who love God all things work together for good, for those who are called according to his purpose." Asking God to reveal His purposes in our pain positions us to view trials through the eyes of faith. Seeing how He is already redeeming the situation for our growth enables bouncing back in hope.

Of course, God's strength is the bedrock beneath our feet when adversity strikes. The prophet Isaiah declared in 40:29, "He gives power to the faint, and to him who has no might he increases strength." Trying to bounce back in our human effort will fall short. But by God's Spirit, we can demonstrate resilient, persevering faith that witnesses to His sustaining grace. May our lives echo Paul's testimony: "We are afflicted in every way, but not crushed...struck down, but not destroyed" (2 Corinthians 4:8-9). Take courage! No adversity can ultimately separate us from the enduring love of Christ.

Understanding the Spirit of Lukewarmness

One of the most dangerous threats to a vibrant faith is the gradual slide into spiritual lukewarmness. Jesus Himself warned the Laodicean church in Revelation 3:15-16, "I know your deeds, that you are neither cold nor hot. I wish you were either one or the other. So, because you are lukewarm, neither hot nor cold, I am about to spit you out of my mouth." What causes this drifting from wholehearted devotion to apathetic religion? How can we recognise and resist the spirit of lukewarmness?

At its root, lukewarmness stems from complacency - believing we have "arrived" spiritually and no longer require zeal, growth, or sacrifice. Pride convinces us that maintenance of the status quo is sufficient. We make following Jesus about clutching what we have rather than pursuing Christ wholeheartedly. But faith requires continually laying down our agendas to embrace His. Lukewarm religion is just going through motions. Lukewarmness also seeps in subtly through neglecting spiritual disciplines. Less time in God's Word, prayer, biblical community, worship, and service to others opens the door to apathy. Just as any relationship decays without intentional investment, our walk with Christ erodes when we stop cultivating intimacy with Him. Is our schedule too full for the practices that fuel the spiritual fire?

Relatedly, refusing correction from godly sources indicates a slide into self-reliance and closed-mindedness - both bedfellows of lukewarmness. Solomon warned in Proverbs 15:32, "He who ignores discipline despises himself, but whoever heeds correction gains understanding." Dodging accountability and biblical counsel keeps us from examining our lives and repenting of sin or compromise. Defensiveness reveals pride in disguise. Additionally, complacency toward fellowship with other believers can breed spiritual lethargy. The book of Hebrews warns in 10:25, "Not neglecting to meet together, as is the habit of some, but encouraging one another, and all the more as you see the Day drawing near." God designed us for the community, and withdrawal shortcircuits His intention. Are we missing out on mutual sharpening and care?

Of course, pursuing lesser affections over loving Christ Himself is lukewarmness at its root. James 4:4 warns, "You adulterous people! Do you not know that friendship with the world is enmity with God?" Divided hearts cannot remain on fire for the Lord. What rivals are we allowing to supplant supreme devotion to Jesus slowly? Idols come in subtle packages. Thankfully, Scripture provides the antidote. Jesus counsels the lukewarm Laodiceans to return to their first love and "be zealous and repent" (Revelation 3:19). We must examine our hearts, ask God to rekindle the spiritual fire, and repent from whatever has promoted creeping complacency. Determine today to give no ground to this dangerous spirit of lukewarmness. Our God deserves a passionate, enduring pursuit of intimacy with Him. May our lives resound, "For me to live is Christ!"

Strategies for Overcoming Spiritual Stagnation

It's easy in our fast-paced, technology-saturated world to drift into spiritual complacency and deadness. Busyness crowds out intentional pursuit of Christ. Distractions bombard our attention span. Before we know it, we exchange an intimate walk with Jesus for a religious routine. How can we recognise and break free from stagnancy? What practical strategies rekindle passion for God?

I will encourage you always to examine your life for symptoms of stagnancy, decreased hunger for God's Word, lack of zeal in worship, wavering prayer life, diminished concern for the lost, tolerance of sin, and struggles bearing spiritual fruit. As Jesus warned the complacent church in Revelation 2:4-5, "You have forsaken the love you had at first. Consider how far you have fallen! Repent and do the things you did at first." Honest assessment positions us for revival. Also, prioritise extended time seeking God rather than quick devotional snippets. Prolonged prayer, meditating on Scripture, journaling, fasting, and listening for His voice realigns our inward focus. The Psalmist cried, "My soul thirsts for God, for the living God" (Psalm 42:2). Do we crave deep encounters with Christ? Disciplined spiritual pursuit restores this "first love" passion.

Immerse yourself in God's Word to retrain thinking and illuminate sin. Hebrews 4:12 declares, "The word of God is living and active, sharper than any two-edged sword, piercing to the division of soul and of spirit, of joints and of marrow, and discerning the thoughts and intentions of the heart." Scripture powerfully recalibrates our worldview when stagnancy clouds spiritual vision. Feasting on God's truths restores our minds. Surround yourself with passionate believers who will challenge your complacency. Proverbs 27:17 notes, "As iron sharpens iron, so one person sharpens another." The fire of revival often spreads through fellowship, testimony, and mutual encouragement among believers. Shared zeal and accountability help reignite fading faith.

Always endeavour to take inventory of your lifestyle for possible idolatry, putting distance between you and Jesus. 1 John 2:15 warns, "Do not love the world or the things in the world." Prolonged exposure to godless media, friends who quench the Spirit, or pleasures crowding out eternal priorities will erode spiritual vigour. Eliminate distractions blocking wholehearted devotion. Most importantly, cry out to the Holy Spirit for fresh fire. Only His power can awaken cold hearts, as David pleaded in Psalm 51:10-11, "Create in me a clean heart, O God, and renew a right spirit within me. Cast me not away from your presence, and take not your Holy Spirit from me. Restore to me the joy of your salvation." Release all to Jesus, asking Him to blaze within you again!

Beloved, stagnancy need not be permanent if we humble ourselves and yield to the Refiner's fire. Jesus promised in Revelation 3:20, "Behold, I stand at the door and knock. If anyone hears my voice and opens the door, I will come into him and eat with him, and he with me." Revival awaits all who make room for Christ again to reign freely. He desires your spiritual fervency, not complacent religion. Draw near to God, and He will rekindle your heart! The best days can be ahead.

The Antidote Lack of Passion

It can be disheartening when we feel cold or lack passion for our pursuit of God. However, we must remember that spiritual fervency is not a constant state, and it is natural to experience ebbs and flows in our journey of faith. The important thing is to acknowledge and address these moments of spiritual apathy, seeking the antidote of repentance to reignite our passion for God and His purposes.

Here are some practical steps to help overcome spiritual coldness and stay fervent:

Recognise and Reflect: The first step in overcoming spiritual coldness is recognising and acknowledging its presence. Take the time to reflect on your spiritual journey and identify the areas where you may have become cold or disconnected from God. This self-awareness will enable you to pinpoint the root causes and take appropriate action.
Seek God's Presence: Prayer is a powerful tool to reconnect with God. Set aside dedicated time to seek His presence. Pour out your heart to Him, confess any sins or areas of complacency, and ask Him to revive your passion for Him. As Psalms 51:10 says, "Create in me a clean heart, O God; and renew a right spirit within me."

Repentance and Surrender: Repentance is the key to restoring our relationship with God. It involves turning away from our sinful actions or attitudes and turning towards God. Repentance requires genuine humility and a willingness to submit to God's will. As we confess our shortcomings and yield to His leadership, He can revitalise our spiritual fervour.

Dive into the Word: The Bible is a source of life and inspiration. Dive into Scripture, read and meditate on God's Word daily. Allow it to convict, encourage, and challenge you. As Hebrews 4:12 reminds us, "For the word of God is quick and powerful, and sharper than any two-edged sword." The more we immerse ourselves in God's Word, the more we experience His transformation in our lives.

Engage in Worship: Worship is a powerful way to connect with God and experience His presence. Whether through singing, praying, or simply surrendering our hearts in adoration, worship helps to shift our focus from ourselves to God. It helps us to remember His goodness, faithfulness, and worthiness of our praise. Our hearts can be reignited as we worship with a deep desire to know Him more.

Fellowship with Believers: Surround yourself with a community of believers who can encourage, inspire, and hold you accountable. Participate in small groups, attend church services, and engage in meaningful conversations with fellow Christians. Iron sharpens iron, and being in the company of other passionate believers can help reignite your zeal for God.

Serve Others: Look for opportunities to serve and bless others. Serving others helps us shift our focus away from ourselves and redirect our attention to the needs of those around us. As we serve selflessly, we experience the joy of being Christ's hands and feet in this world. It strengthens our faith and reminds us of the purpose of our calling.

Cultivate a Spirit of Gratitude: Develop an attitude of gratitude for all that God has done and continues to do in your life. Focus on His blessings, His faithfulness, and His provisions. Expressing gratitude shifts our perspective and helps us see God's hand in our lives. Gratitude paves the way for a renewed passion and love for God.

Remember, staying fervent in our pursuit of God is a lifelong journey. It is normal to experience seasons of coldness, but with repentance and a desire to draw close to

God, we can overcome and find renewed fervency. Trust in God's grace and rely on His strength to sustain you on this journey of faith. May your heart be set ablaze with passion as you seek after God's heart and purpose for your life.

Examining Heart Motives

In our journey as Christians, examining our heart motives becomes vital in our pursuit of a genuine and fruitful relationship with God. Our motives reflect the intentions behind our actions and reveal the state of our hearts. As believers, it is crucial that our motives align with God's intentions, demonstrating a sincere desire to please Him and bless others. The Bible urges us to examine our motives and ensure they are rooted in pure and selfless intentions. Let us explore the significance of sincere motives before God and men and how they lead to ultimate rewards. Our motives speak volumes about who we are as individuals and disciples of Christ. They are the driving force behind our actions and determine the outcomes we experience. Proverbs 16:2 states, "All the ways of a man are clean in his own eyes; but the Lord weigheth the spirits." This verse reminds us that while we may perceive our actions as righteous, God truly examines our hearts' motivations. Therefore, we must consciously and honestly evaluate our motives to ensure they align with God's intentions.

First and foremost, our motives should be centred on pleasing and glorifying God. As Christians, our primary goal is to honour Him in all that we do. 1 Corinthians 10:31 states, "Whether, therefore, ye eat, or drink, or whatsoever ye do, do all to the glory of God." This verse highlights the all-encompassing nature of our motive, urging us to align every aspect of our lives to bring glory to God. When our motives are rooted in genuine love for God and a desire to obey His commands, we experience true transformation and deepen our relationship with Him.

Furthermore, our motives should also extend to our relationships with others. Jesus Himself instructed us to love one another and serve others selflessly. Matthew 22:39 states, "And the second [commandment] is like unto it; thou shalt love thy neighbour as thyself." Our motives in our interactions with others should be driven by sincere love and a desire to bless rather than seeking personal gain or recognition. When we genuinely care for and serve others with pure motives, we reflect the love of Christ and become instruments of His grace and mercy.

It is important to note that while we should strive to have pure motives, we are inherently flawed and capable of self-serving intentions. Our motives can become tainted by pride, selfishness, and seeking personal rewards. However, when we surrender our hearts to God and allow Him to transform us, He can purify our motives and align them with His divine purposes. Psalm 51:10 says, "Create in me a clean heart, O God; and renew a right spirit within me." This verse expresses a humble plea for God's cleansing and renewal, acknowledging our need for His intervention in our motives. When our motives align with God's intentions, it brings about various rewards. These rewards may not always be material or immediate, but they are of eternal significance. God is concerned with our external actions and the state of our hearts. He rewards those who diligently seek Him and serve others with sincerity. James 4:8 affirms this, saying, "Draw nigh to God, and he will draw nigh to you." When our motives align with God's desires, we experience a deeper sense of His presence, guidance, and peace.

Moreover, our motives influence our impact on others and the legacy we leave behind. When we genuinely serve and love others, they witness the transformational power of Christ in us. Our motives can inspire and encourage others to seek God and live with sincerity in their own lives. Our lives become a testament to God's grace and love, impacting those around us and pointing them towards the ultimate reward of eternal life in Christ. So, examining our heart motives is vital in our Christian walk. Our motives should be centred on pleasing and glorifying God and serving others selflessly. While we may sometimes struggle with self-serving motives, surrendering our hearts to God allows Him to purify and align our motives with His divine purposes. When our motives are sincere and aligned with God's intentions, we experience His rewards through a deeper relationship with Him, a meaningful impact on others, and the assurance of eternal blessings. Let us continually evaluate our motives, seeking God's guidance and grace to ensure they reflect His desires for our lives.

Learning from Failure and Avoiding the Next Occurrence

Failure is an inevitable part of life, and as Christians, we are not exempt from experiencing setbacks and disappointments. However, what sets us apart is our response to failure. Instead of being defined by our failures, we have the opportunity to learn from them and grow in our faith. Scripture provides us with guidance on how to navigate failure, offering wisdom and encouragement to avoid repeat occurrences. Let us explore the importance of learning from failure and the steps we can take to avoid repeating past mistakes. Failure can be a humbling experience, revealing our weaknesses and limitations. It is an opportunity for introspection and growth. Proverbs 24:16 says, "For a just man falleth seven times, and riseth up again: but the wicked shall fall into mischief." This verse reminds us that even as righteous individuals, we may encounter failure, but what matters is our ability to rise up and keep moving forward. When we approach our failures with humility and a desire to learn, we allow God to work in us and teach us valuable lessons.

Learning from failure requires a genuine self-reflection and a willingness to take responsibility for our actions. Instead of blaming others or external circumstances, we must examine our choices and attitudes. Psalm 139:23-24 says, "Search me, O God, and know my heart: try me, and know my thoughts: And see if there be any wicked way in me and lead me in the way everlasting." This verse encourages us to invite God into the process of examining our hearts and thoughts, allowing Him to reveal any areas of wrongdoing or sinful patterns. When we take ownership of our failures, we open ourselves up to God's correction and guidance. After reflecting on our failures, seeking God's forgiveness and embracing His grace is important. Failure does not define us as Christians; it is an opportunity for growth and transformation. Through the sacrifice of Jesus Christ, we have been offered forgiveness for our failures and the hope of a fresh start. Romans 8:1 reassures us, "There is, therefore, now no condemnation to them which are in Christ Jesus, who walk not after the flesh, but after the Spirit." God's grace empowers us to move beyond our failures and strive for righteousness.

We must learn from and make intentional changes to avoid repeating past mistakes. This requires developing a discerning spirit and seeking wisdom from God. Proverbs 3:5-6 advises, "Trust in the LORD with all thine heart; and lean not unto thine own understanding. In all thy ways acknowledge him, and he shall direct thy paths." By trusting in God's guidance and seeking His wisdom, we can make informed decisions and avoid falling into the same pitfalls. Surrendering ourselves to God's leading enables us to break free from destructive patterns and pursue a life of obedience and purpose. It is also beneficial to seek counsel and accountability from fellow believers. Proverbs 11:14 states, "Where no counsel is, the people fall: but in the multitude of counsellors there is safety." Connecting with wise and trustworthy individuals who can offer guidance and hold us accountable can help prevent us from repeating past mistakes. Together, we can encourage and support one another in our pursuit of godliness.

In a nutshell, as Christians, we have the privilege of learning from failure and avoiding repeat occurrences. Approaching failure with humility and a desire to learn allows us to grow in our faith and character. Through self-reflection, seeking forgiveness and embracing God's grace, we can move forward with the lessons learned from our failures. By trusting in God's guidance, seeking wisdom, and embracing accountability, we can make informed decisions and avoid falling into the same traps. Let us remember that failure does not define us, but rather, it is an opportunity for God's transformative work in our lives.

Chapter 5

Revelation 3v2 - A Call to Overcome Lukewarmness

One of Jesus' most sobering warnings comes in His letter to the church in Laodicea, who He rebukes for lukewarm faith and calls for repentance. Revelation 3:2 records Christ's confrontation of their spiritual apathy: "I know your works, that you are neither cold nor hot. I could wish you were cold or hot. So then, because you are lukewarm and neither cold nor hot, I will vomit you out of My mouth." What vital lessons can we apply from this firm caution against creeping complacency?

Jesus clarifies that being "neither cold nor hot," stuck between half-hearted religion and wholehearted surrender, provokes disgust from Him. Lukewarmness reflects distasteful indifference concerning growth, obedience, and intimacy with Christ. It is the temperature of compromised faith that mixes worldly thinking with biblical truth. Our Lord desires fiery, passionate pursuit above all else. Does He detect division of affection in us?

Lukewarmness does not happen overnight but is the result of drifting gradually. Earlier in Revelation 2:4, Jesus rebuked Ephesus, saying, "You have left your first love." As with any relationship, our affections cool through taking our eyes off Christ to focus on other priorities. We must frequently evaluate the thermometer of loyalty to Him versus culture or comfort. Are you as awestruck by His glory as when first saved? Christ's stern warning to Laodicea reveals that lukewarmness grieves the heart of God. Jesus laments, "I wish you were cold or hot." Coldness is at least an honest rejection versus claiming His name while apathetically keeping Him at arm's length. Let this serve as a sobering reminder that we are called to earnestly "press toward the mark for the prize of the high calling of God in Christ Jesus" (Philippians 3:14), not religious complacency. Does our lifestyle reflect the wholehearted pursuit of Jesus?

Scripture gives hope that revived passion is possible through repentance. Jesus continues in Revelation 3:19: "Those whom I love, I reprove and discipline, so be zealous and repent." We all are prone to wander at times. But as we humbly receive the Lord's correction, embrace conviction, and return to our first love, He eagerly reconciles and restores the fire of devotion. Do you need to heed His warning call to repent from lukewarmness? He stands ready to revive the contrite heart. At this stage, this passage reminds us that only the Spirit's empowerment sustains lifelong fervency. Trying to rekindle the passion for human strength will fail. But as we yield control of every area to the Lordship of Jesus, He fans into flame a spiritual zeal that withstands seasons of dryness or doubt. May our prayer echo Paul's in Galatians 2:20, "I have been crucified with Christ. It is no longer I who live, but Christ who lives in me." He is faithful in completing the work He began in us (Philippians 1:6). Beloved, stay true to your first Love.

Exploring the Scripture and Its Relevance

The Bible makes bold claims about itself that compel us to examine its pages closely. 2 Timothy 3:16-17 declares, "All Scripture is breathed out by God and profitable for teaching, for reproof, for correction, and for training in righteousness, that the man of God may be complete, equipped for every good work." What does it mean that these writings are "God-breathed"? How did we receive the remarkable gift of Holy Scripture, and why is it utterly unique among books? Foremost, the Bible affirms that its words originated not from human initiative but from the very mouth of God. Over 40 authors, writing over 1500 years in different languages and cultures, penned God's messages according to His timing and promptings. Though they employed their own styles, personalities, and vocabularies, the Spirit of God moved upon these men to record His flawless, eternal words through them (2 Peter 1:20-21). Scripture came not "by the will of man, but of God."

Also, biblical authors were eyewitnesses to the events they recorded by God's inspiration. John opens his first epistle, declaring, "That which was from the beginning, which we have heard, which we have seen with our eyes, which we looked upon and have touched with our hands...we also proclaim to you" (1 John 1:1,3). Luke states his gospel was compiled from firsthand research and testimony (Luke 1:1-4). Moses participated personally in Israel's wilderness wanderings, which he chronicled. The Bible was grounded in actual history. Scripture emphasizes that no part of itself originates from private interpretation or prophecy but from direct revelation by the Holy Spirit. Peter attests that "the will of man ever produced no prophecy, but men spoke from God as they were carried along by the Holy

Spirit" (2 Peter 1:20-21). The prophets and apostles received and recorded the pure oracles of God as His Spirit enabled them. Scripture comes directly from heaven's throne.

Why is acknowledging Scripture's divine inspiration crucial? When we recognize the Bible as God's authentic, authoritative voice, we receive it as our sole trustworthy guide for doctrine, reproof, correction, and righteous living (2 Timothy 3:16-17). Scripture alone stands as the compass pointing us to salvation and discernment amidst competing voices. It is the Father's love letter beckoning us to know His heart and purposes. Are we anchored wholly to this eternal Word? Despite the rise and fall of cultures, philosophies, and human understanding, God's truth remains unchanged and relevant. "The grass withers and the flower falls, but the word of the Lord remains forever" (1 Peter 1:24-25). May our lives be rooted and guided by these holy writings breathed out by the Spirit of the living God. Just as Jesus used Scripture to thwart temptation (Matthew 4:1-11), may the Bible light our path until we see our Savior face to face. It alone is "a lamp unto our feet and light unto our path" (Psalm 119:105).

Applying the Message to Modern Spiritual Challenges

Amidst an ever-shifting culture, the timeless truths of Scripture provide steadfast guidance, wisdom and correction for navigating the complexities of modern life. The same Holy Spirit who inspired the biblical authors continues illuminating its principles for our current times. As Paul wrote in 2 Timothy 3:16-17, "All Scripture is breathed out by God and profitable for teaching, for reproof, for correction, and training in righteousness, that the man of God may be competent, equipped for every good work." How do we faithfully apply the Bible's life-giving message to the spiritual challenges of today?

We must approach Scripture expecting God to speak with relevance in specific situations. His Word is "living and active" (Hebrews 4:12), intended to pierce hearts in every generation and culture. As we open the Bible, pray for the Spirit to make its teachings leap from page to life with personalized direction. Ask the Lord to illuminate your circumstances through the lens of biblical truth, replacing human reasoning with heavenly insight. Consider writing down Scripture verses that speak to your current struggles and decisions to meditate on throughout the day.

Learn to saturate your mind with Scripture to gain perspective for applying it. Psalm 1:1-3 describes the blessed man as one who delights in God's law, meditating on it day and night. Immersing our minds in the Bible renews our thinking to align with the mind of Christ. Biblical truth informs our reflex responses to situations. When facing conflicts, struggles, ethical dilemmas and decisions, Scriptural principles embedded in our hearts rise to guide our conduct and become a compass for wise application.

Rely on the Spirit's power rather than willpower to obey Scripture. We often fail in applying God's Word through depending on human effort alone. But as Zechariah 4:6 declares, "'Not by might, nor by power, but by My Spirit,' says the LORD of hosts." Pray for the Holy Spirit to empower you towards obedience. He is the Spirit of truth who inspired Scripture and alone can produce its fruit in our lives (John 14:17, John 15:5). Our part is yielding wholeheartedly to Him; His role is transforming us increasingly into Christlikeness.

Put Scripture's teachings into practice through accountable relationships and church community. We gain wisdom on applying God's Word well through the Body of Christ (Proverbs 15:22, Proverbs 27:17). Whether through a mentor, small group, or pastor, trusted fellow believers help us appropriately live out the Bible's commands. For example, when struggling with an unforgiving spirit, sharing this vulnerability within the Christian community can lead to bearing one another's burdens (Galatians 6:2), prayer support, and practical Scriptural counsel on walking in grace. Accountability helps prevent misapplying Scripture.

In all of it, test all counsel and decision-making against the plumb line of Scripture. God's Word is the ultimate authority and filter for evaluating life choices and situations. Rather than reacting based on emotions or human wisdom, we must continually ask, "What does the Bible say about this?" Scripture provides clear morals on matters of integrity. When facing major decisions like jobs or relationships, biblical principles on seeking God's will direct our steps. God's unchanging truths call the shots - not fluctuating culture.

On a personal note, a timely example from my life involves leaving a demanding job compromising important priorities. Biblical Sabbath rest principles, wisdom on seasons and priorities from Ecclesiastes, and trusted friends' counsel all pointed to releasing this role to focus on more urgent callings from the Lord for this phase of life. Applying Scriptural guidance with Spirit empowerment led to freedom, peace, and new opportunities I'm now embracing. May our lives evidence the blessedness of building upon the enduring rock of God's Word! Amidst the shifting sands of modern culture, applying biblical truth with wisdom, discernment and the Spirit's help anchors our lives to what truly matters now and for eternity.

Navigating Moral Dilemmas

In our fallen world, followers of Christ inevitably encounter situations where biblical values clash with cultural norms or self-interest. How do we navigate moral grey areas to make wise choices pleasing to God? When faced with difficult dilemmas, several biblical principles can guide our response.

First, bathe the decision in prayer, asking God for wisdom and moral clarity. James 1:5 promises, "If any of you lacks wisdom, let him ask God, who gives generously to all without reproach, and it will be given him." Bringing dilemmas before the Lord aligns our hearts with His values and illuminates blind spots we cannot see. As Psalm 25:4-5 declares, "Make me to know your ways, O Lord; teach me your paths. Lead me in your truth and teach me." God promises to guide the humble seeker.

Examine any potential choice through the lens of Scripture. Hebrews 4:12 says God's word is "sharper than any two-edged sword, piercing to the division of soul and of spirit, of joints and of marrow, and discerning the thoughts and intentions of the heart." Applying biblical principles helps cut through murky inner motives to discern righteousness from rationalization. Does our decision align with truths like loving others, submitting to governing authorities, speaking with integrity, and avoiding evil appearances?

Seek wise counsel from mature believers. Proverbs 11:14 warns that "in an abundance of counsellors there is safety." God often provides perspective through a thoughtful friend or pastor who can identify blind spots. As Proverbs 27:17 notes, "Iron sharpens iron, and one man sharpens another." Voice concerns and listen humbly to outside input. The multiplicity of counsel provides a fuller understanding.

Consider any precedent or influence the choice could set. Paul cautions in 1 Corinthians 8:9, "Take care that this right of yours does not somehow become a stumbling block to the weak." While an action may not be expressly forbidden, it could open the door for moral compromise down the road or cause a weaker brother to stumble. Weigh potential long-term consequences on oneself or others.

Evaluate the decision in light of God's purposes for your life. 1 Corinthians 10:31 challenges believers, "So, whether you eat or drink, or whatever you do, do all to the glory of God." Will this action glorify the Lord and align with the good works He prepared for me, or distract and detract? Stewarding our decisions well maximizes kingdom impact. Above all, let love for God and others guide your moral reasoning. Jesus taught that the entire law hangs on the greatest commandments - to love the Lord with all your heart, soul, mind and strength, and love your neighbour as yourself (Matthew 22:37-39). Analyzing dilemmas through the lens of agape love keeps our choices rooted in care for people, not selfish interests.

With much prayer, wisdom, and reliance on the Spirit's guidance, believers can navigate murky moral waters in keeping with God's purposes. Though difficult dilemmas will arise, we have every resource needed to choose what honours Christ. As Colossians 1:9-10 declares, "We have not ceased to pray for you, asking that you may be filled with the knowledge of his will in all spiritual wisdom and understanding, so as to walk in a manner worthy of the Lord, fully pleasing to him." He will illuminate the path as we seek His face.

Chapter 6
Embracing the Unfinished Work of God

As Christ's followers, we are stewards of a holy yet unfinished work spanning generations, furthering God's Kingdom on earth before Jesus returns. Though we cannot finish the task, Scripture exhorts us to embrace the sacred privilege of contributing to the Great Commission across our lifetimes. Just as esteemed forefathers and foremothers of faith ran their laps well, the baton now passes to our hands. How do we take up the unfinished work of God with endurance and passion worthy of our calling?

We must live with open hands, acknowledging that our lives belong fully to God for His purposes. Paul reminds believers in 1 Corinthians 6:19-20, "You are not your own, for you were bought with a price." Our time, resources, gifts, and talents are not ours to control, but ultimately, it is His to invest where He chooses. Dying to selfish ambition and personal comfort frees us to use all we are for God's glory. Abandonment to the King will propel the building of a selfless kingdom. Cultivating intimacy with Christ fuels work rooted in relationship rather than duty. Jesus said in John 15:5, "I am the vine; you are the branches. Whoever abides in me and I in him, he is that bears much fruit, for apart from me, you can do nothing." As Hudson Taylor wrote, "All God's giants were weak men who did great things for God because they reckoned on His power and presence with them." Fruitfulness flows from abiding, not human striving. The work lasts when He works through us.

We must see ourselves as continuers of an unfinished story authored by God alone. Hebrews 12:1 reminds us we are "surrounded by so great a cloud of witnesses." Saints have gone before us for centuries, playing their part. But there are more chapters yet to be written before Christ's return. We steward but a page in the epic narrative of God building His Kingdom on earth as it is in heaven. This should produce holy urgency amidst short life spans.

Guide against not finishing; finishing the work requires running together in a community, not independent of fellow labourers. Ecclesiastes 4:9 states, "Two are better than one because they have a good reward for their toil." The diversity of Christ's body ensures all necessary gifts are operating. We gain strength, wisdom and accountability to persevere when joining hands, resources and anointings with trusted Kingdom companions. Only together can we maximize our reach. Excelling in unfinished work means constantly passing the baton to emerging generations. Paul poured tirelessly into his young disciple Timothy, charging him to entrust Christ's truths to faithful messengers who would carry it forward (2 Timothy 2:2). We are stewards of a sacred trust, responsible for reproducing fruit that remains. This requires identifying, mentoring and empowering younger believers to shoulder tomorrow's challenges.

In a nutshell, only the empowerment of the Holy Spirit enables finishing the race with passion. Zechariah 4:6 says, "'Not by might, nor by power, but by my Spirit,' says the Lord of hosts." You and I will inevitably fall short;

thankfully, weakness makes His strength perfect. Leaning wholly on the Spirit who conceived the work spurs us on. Managing unfinished tasks can wait; may our life's singular passion be knowing and obeying Jesus. On a personal level, for years, I viewed my work primarily as ticking tasks off a to-do list. I tended to define productivity solely by visible results while neglecting the central priority of abiding in Christ. The Lord convinced me through His word and wise counsel that ministry fruitfulness flows from intimacy with Him. My role is staying connected to the True Vine amidst labour. This renewed perspective on the unfinished work of God as His story - not mine - has profoundly shaped my priorities and peace. Outcomes rest in His hands as I walk faithfully with Him day by precious day.

What honour we have been given as stewards of the Highest God's unfinished symphony. With the radiant hope of eternity secure, let us give our fleeting days on earth to further His Kingdom with wholehearted devotion. "Let us run with endurance the race that is set before us, looking to Jesus, the founder and perfecter of our faith" (Hebrews 12:1-2). May the Master find us faithful when we rest from our labours. The work He began, He will complete.

God's Perspective on Human Accomplishments

Our culture fixates on external markers of achievement, wealth, fame, accolades, and image. But biblical truth reveals our human status symbols as fleeting vanity from God's eternal viewpoint. 1 Samuel 16:7 declares, "Man looks at the outward appearance, but the LORD looks at the heart." How does our Creator assess and measure lives differently than worldly scales of success? What pursuits hold value in His kingdom economy? While society elevates pride and self-reliance, God opposes the proud but gives grace to the humble (James 4:6). Jesus pronounced blessings on the poor in spirit, the meek, the merciful, and the pure in heart (Matthew 5:3-8) - those who recognize their spiritual bankruptcy apart from Him. While the world bows to the ambitious go-getter, our Lord lifts up the soul contrite and dependent upon His strength alone. Kingdom impact flows from humility, not skill.

Likewise, God values inward integrity, not outward jewellery or status, as in 1 Peter 3:3-4: "Do not let your adorning be external...but let your adorning be the hidden person of the heart." While humankind fixates on exteriors, the Lord examines hearts. Any good deeds or ministry fruit not flowing from inner communion with Christ count as worthless before Him. Only that which springs from abiding in the Vine holds eternal weight. The Lord measures life not in years but in faithfulness and obedience. As Jesus said in John 15:16, "You did not choose me, but I chose you and appointed you that you should go and bear fruit and that your fruit should abide." Our call is simply to walk in step with His Spirit, leaving impact results to the Master. Some plant, some water, but God gives the increase in His timing (1 Corinthians 3:6-7). Staying faithful to our particular mission matters more than visible outcomes we can tally.

In addition, God values servanthood, not high position. Jesus warned His disciples against emulating worldly authority, saying, "Whoever desires to become great among you shall be your servant" (Matthew 20:26). The path to true greatness ascends downward in laying down rights and serving others, just as our Lord demonstrated. Heaven's hierarchy differs drastically from earthly importance. Our worth is not measured by the prominence of our role but by the humility and love shown. The Lord weighs our work by eternal versus earthly gain. Paul wrote in 1 Corinthians 3:13-14, "Each one's work will become clear; for the Day will declare it because it will be revealed by fire; and the fire will test each one's work, of what sort it is." All our labour will be evaluated to see whether it was built on Christ versus worldly wisdom. Only "gold, silver, precious stones" refined in the fire of the Spirit's transforming work will stand. Does our effort aim for imperishable gains?

As beloved children of our Abba Father, may we find identity and purpose not in chasing worldly trophies but in pursuing the loving approval of our Lord. When we live to bring a smile to the face of God alone, obeying His voice with childlike devotion, then we store up treasures in heaven that will endure forever. Our life accomplishments fade to ashes minus God. But a heart abandoned fully to Jesus emerges as gold tested and refined for His glory.

Living with Purpose in Light of Unfinished Business

As followers of Jesus, we are stewards of an immense, unfinished work, expanding God's kingdom on earth before Christ returns. Though we cannot complete this cosmic task, we are called to embrace our sacred role of furthering His plans during our finite lifetimes. But how do we stay focused on our mission when unfinished goals and unresolved matters tempt us toward discouragement? What empowers purposeful living amidst imperfection?

Foremost, remembering that our labour is part of a much greater story lifts us above life's interruptions. Paul declares in 1 Corinthians 3:9, "For we are God's fellow workers." All we do to advance His gospel contributes to a timeless, sovereign plan spanning millennia. Our unfinished work is a thread in a grand tapestry only He can view. This big-picture perspective steadies us during seasons of interruption or delay. No effort in Him is wasted, regardless of closure. Entrusting outcomes to God's timing grants patience to persevere. Ecclesiastes 3:11 reminds us, "He has made everything beautiful in its time." The Master Craftsman oversees projects in process with perfect understanding. Some spiritual seeds take decades to sprout; others, we will only see fruit from in eternity. Faithfulness matters more than complete resolution. Walking in step with the Spirit and leaving results to Him lightens the burden of unfinished work.

Excelling in present phases sharpens focus against comparing ourselves to others. Paul charges in Galatians 6:4, "But let each one examine his own work, and then he will have to rejoice in himself alone and not in another." Staying in our lane, improving our skills, and finishing what's on our plates today poises us for expanded responsibilities tomorrow. We each contribute through unique callings. Comparing breeds discontentment; contentment fuels purpose. Unfinished business is God's invitation to trust His strength over our inadequacy. Paul said in 2 Corinthians 12:9, "My grace is sufficient for you, for my power is made perfect in weakness." When we feel overwhelmed by the work's scope, God reminds us that the battle belongs to Him. Our part is showing up with yielded hearts. Zechariah 4:6 promises, "'Not by might nor by power, but by my Spirit,' says the Lord." Leaning wholly on divine empowerment liberates us to live purposefully in the midst of imperfection.

We must view unfinished work as intended for equipping others to shoulder. Paul told Timothy in 2 Timothy 2:2, "What you have heard from me...entrust to faithful men who will be able to teach others also." The work is a living legacy spanning generations. Our responsibility is to develop more labourers, not personally tie up loose ends. Multiplying impact through mentorship is key to finishing well. Passing the baton also reminds us that our part in God's story is but one chapter. Future saints will write more. Above all, purpose amidst imperfection flows from an identity rooted in Christ, not our unfinished tasks. As Paul declares in Philippians 3:8-9, everything else pales beside "the surpassing worth of knowing Christ Jesus my Lord." When we find supreme acceptance and delight in Him, we stop striving and rest in His love. Our calling is not checking off items but pursuing intimacy with Jesus daily. Abiding in the Vine enables fruitfulness. May unfinished work drive us closer to the One who completes us.

As servants of the Highest God, may we stay invested as stewards with patience and endurance while leaving outcomes to the Master? Despite interruptions and imperfections, we can live purposefully by remembering our role in God's greater plan. By His strength and for His glory, we will bear eternal fruit as we walk faithfully with Him day by precious day. Our labour in the Lord is never in vain.

Finishing Well

My dear brothers and sisters in Christ, as we traverse the path of life, we are often consumed by the desire to achieve success and leave a lasting legacy. We pour our energy into pursuing our dreams, whether they be personal or professional, and strive to make a difference in the world. However, amidst these pursuits, it is imperative that we never lose sight of an even greater aspiration to finish well in our faith journey. The concept of finishing well is deeply rooted in the teachings of the Bible. Throughout the scriptures, we find stories of individuals who faced trials, tribulations, and temptations but remained steadfast in their commitment to God. Their perseverance in the face of adversity sets a powerful example for us to follow.

One such example is the apostle Paul. In his letter to the Corinthians, he writes, "I have fought a good fight, I have finished my course, I have kept the faith" (2 Timothy 4:7). These words embody the essence of finishing well - a relentless determination to stay true to our beliefs until the very end. Paul's life serves as a testament to the transformative power of God's grace, even in the face of persecution and hardship. Another inspiring figure from the Bible is Job. Despite losing everything he held dear, Job remained faithful to God. In the end, God restored his fortunes and blessed him abundantly. Job teaches us that finishing well is about achieving personal success and trusting in God's plan and purpose for our lives. As we go through seasons of struggle and loss, we must cling to our faith, knowing that God is still at work and will bring about a glorious outcome.

So, how do we finish well in our own lives? It starts with cultivating a deep and intimate relationship with God. Just as a thriving plant needs regular nourishment, our spiritual lives require a consistent and intentional connection with our Heavenly Father. Through prayer, Bible study, and fellowship with other believers, we can draw closer to God and gain the wisdom and strength to persevere. In addition, finishing well requires a commitment to spiritual discipline. It is not enough to simply believe in God; we must also live out our faith daily. This means walking in love, pursuing holiness, and serving others selflessly. Jesus reminds us, "But he that shall endure unto the end, the same shall be saved." (Matthew 24:13). Our faith is not a one-time event but a lifelong journey, and it is through our actions that we demonstrate our commitment to finishing well.

Also, embracing a humble and teachable spirit is crucial to finishing well. We must be willing to learn and grow, allowing God to refine and mould us into the likeness of Christ. As the apostle Peter writes, "But grow in grace, and in the knowledge of our Lord and Savior Jesus Christ" (2 Peter 3:18). This continuous pursuit of growth and transformation ensures that we never become stagnant or complacent in our faith. So, finishing well requires us to fix our gaze on the ultimate prize, eternity with God. In the grand scheme of things, our earthly accomplishments and accolades pale in comparison to the eternal glory that awaits us. As Paul writes to the Philippians, "I press toward the mark for the prize of the high calling of God in Christ Jesus" (Philippians 3:14). Our journey of faith is not just about the here and now; it is about the everlasting joy and fulfillment that will be ours in God's presence.

My dear brothers and sisters, as we navigate the challenges and uncertainties of life, let us fix our eyes on Jesus, the author and finisher of our faith (Hebrews 12:2). Let us stand firm in our commitment to finishing well, knowing that God is faithful and will equip us with everything we need to persevere. May we be found faithful till the end, bringing glory to His name and inspiring others to walk this same path of faith. Remember, dear friends, finishing well is not easy, but it is worth every effort and sacrifice. Through the grace of God, we can overcome every obstacle and finish our race with unwavering faith. As we embark on this journey together, let us encourage and uplift one another, spurring each other towards the ultimate goal - to hear our Heavenly Father say, "Well done, thou good and faithful servant" (Matthew 25:23).

May the Lord bless you and keep you, even as we finish well and strong.

Chapter 7

The Continuous Journey of Personal Growth

As followers of Christ, spiritual growth is not a one-time event but a lifelong process. Until the day we meet Jesus face to face, there is always room for progress in reflecting more of His character and purpose. What mindsets and practices enable ongoing personal development into maturity? How do we maintain fresh eyes to see areas needing growth?

Humility and teachability are essential for continuous improvement. Proverbs remind us that "knowledge comes easily to the teachable" (Proverbs 16:21) and "those who listen when corrected will live a full life" (Proverbs 15:31). The moment we think we have arrived, our capacity to grow shuts down. But when we maintain a learner's pliable, humble heart, change remains possible. Do we listen well to correction and seek out perspectives beyond our own?

Connecting regularly with trusted mentors and communities provides a mirror highlighting blind spots we cannot easily see alone. Proverbs 27:17 notes, "As iron sharpens iron, so one person sharpens another." There are lessons revealed through friendship and counsel that would otherwise remain hidden. The refinement of godly accountability helps shape us steadily toward maturity. Are you allowing others to speak into your life?

Staying sensitive to the Spirit's prompting aids our responsiveness to areas needing change. Jesus said the Holy Spirit would guide believers into all truth and convict them of sin and righteousness (John 16:8, 13). As we nurture sensitivity through prayer and Scripture meditation, the Spirit gently reveals attitudes and habits in need of realignment. His whispers prepare us for growth that leads to freedom. Are you attentive to the Spirit's work in your inner life?

Cultivating gratitude, rather than entitlement, fosters ongoing teachability. When we begin expecting ease, appreciation for mentors, hard-won lessons, and progress made dims. Thankfulness acknowledges growth as a gift, not something we earn or control. Gratitude also frees us from bitterness when trials come. Thankful hearts stay receptive to divine sculpting. Are you quick to acknowledge lessons gained and progress made?

Purposefully planting ourselves in places of discomfort moves us toward needed growth. As author Don Miller wrote, "To get to the fruit, you have to go out on the limb." New levels of spiritual maturity often require leaving our comfort zones and embracing unfamiliar change. Learning happens in the stretches. Are there new situations or roles where God may be inviting you to courageously step out and grow?

Keep this in mind, serving the King of kings fosters a high view of the Christian life. Jesus urges his disciples in Luke 12:48, "To whom much is given, much is required." Reverence for the Lord who redeemed us propels a desire to steward our growth well, rather than settling for complacency. A holy God deserves our very best, a lifetime of passionate pursuit. Does your vision of God stir your soul towards greater Christlikeness?

Most importantly, abiding in a loving relationship with Jesus fuels continual transformation. Separate from the Vine, our capacity bears little fruit (John 15:5). But as we feast on Scripture, communicate intimately with the Lord, and centre on His presence through the Spirit, His life flows into and transforms ours. Nearness to Christ is the non-negotiable prerequisite to all lasting growth. Is He your supreme desire and delight? While the process of growth brings occasional growing pains as God chips away at our selfishness, the joy of reflecting on Jesus makes every bit of discomfort worthwhile. Let us embrace the journey with patience, eager expectation, and childlike reliance on the Spirit's help. "Let us...continue to grow in every way more and more like Christ" (Ephesians 4:15). The day we see our Savior face to face, we will realize just how worth all the growth was. Until then, we have the privilege of discovering Him more each step along the way. Our best days are still unfolding.

Emphasizing the Journey over the Destination

In our results-driven world, achieving goals, milestones, and dreams can easily overshadow enjoying the preciousness of each day's journey. Ecclesiastes 3:11 reminds us that God "has made everything beautiful in its time." How can we walk skillfully through life, emphasizing loving God and others well right now versus viewing today as just a means to a destination?

Nurturing daily intimacy with Christ is key to keeping our eyes on the eternal versus temporal. Jesus said in John 15:5, "I am the vine; you are the branches. Whoever abides in me and I in him, he is that bears much fruit, for apart from me, you can do nothing." Apart from daily surrender and communion, it's easy to depend on our strength and neglect abiding in His love. Evaluating each day by our connection with Jesus gives the present moment purpose regardless of "outcomes."

Focusing on obedient consistency in small things loosens the grip of future goal setting. Luke 16:10 says, "One who is faithful in a very little is also faithful in much." God often prepares us for more visible assignments through hidden years of loyal service in small duties. Sacred significance exists in the humble repetitiveness of daily surrender to Christ. Undramatic faithfulness outpaces fleeting achievement.

Embracing seasons of waiting and preparation cultivates patience and trust in God's timing. Psalm 37:7 counsels, "Be still before the Lord and wait patiently for him." The journey is not something to "get through" hastily but a space designed by God to deepen character and intimacy with Him. Understanding the journey's purpose steadies us to walk slowly and attentively with Him through life's deserts and valleys.

Cherishing relationships and memories along the path brings meaning to the journey. Life is enriched by loving well, savouring long talks, knowing others' stories, celebrating milestones, grieving losses, forgiving offences, and bearing one another's burdens. In Ephesians 5:16, Paul urges us to make the most of our time not by rushing but by understanding that life is short and prioritizing people well.

Nurturing an attitude of gratitude savours God's everyday graces versus hurrying past them. 1 Thessalonians 5:18

instructs to "give thanks in all circumstances for this is God's will for you in Christ Jesus." Gratitude notices and honours the holy in humble moments - morning light, bird song, delicious flavours, belly laughs. Train your eyes to admire God's handiwork and gifts surrounding you right where you are. Most importantly, remembering our eternal destination infuses daily steps with a holy purpose. As Paul declares in 2 Corinthians 4:16–18, "We do not lose heart. This light momentary affliction is preparing us an eternal weight of glory." With heaven's hope secure, we can walk patiently through earthly joys and trials, our gaze fixed on Jesus and hearts anchored in our unshakable future with Him.

While goals and plans have their place, the gift lies less in some distant achievement than in who we become along the way. As Dallas Willard wrote, "Hurry is the great enemy of spiritual life." May we walk slowly with Jesus, carefully stewards of each day He gives. The journey was never merely the preface - it is the story itself revealed line upon precious line as we yield to Him. Keep step today, beloved. Our eternal tomorrow awaits, but we have this irreplaceable now.

Cultivating a Mindset of Lifelong Learning

Maintaining a teachable spirit over a lifetime can be countercultural in a culture obsessed with youth. Yet Scripture extols the virtues of lifelong learning, urging followers of Christ to stay hungry students no matter their age or experience. Solomon, the wisest man who ever lived, exhorted, "Listen to advice and accept discipline, and at the end you will be counted among the wise" (Proverbs 19:20). What mindsets and habits nurture continuous growth? How do we fight complacency?

First, humility is essential for lifelong learning. Proverbs teaches, "Fools think their own way is right, but the wise listen to others" (Proverbs 12:15). A know-it-all attitude stunts growth, but humility acknowledges that we all have blind spots. Approaching life like a child—curious, eager, receptive to correction—keeps our hearts soft and moldable. Do we listen well, ask sincere questions, and receive feedback without defensiveness? Pride calcifies minds against change.

Secondly, viewing life itself as a classroom cultivates lifelong learning. Paul discovered contentment in all circumstances by adapting to life's curveballs, saying, "I have learned the secret of being content in any and every situation" (Philippians 4:12). If we believe every experience offers potential wisdom to apply, disappointment or detours become valuable lessons. Asking, "What is this trying to teach me?" positions us to learn from all of life.

Additionally, cross-generational relationships expand understanding and combat civil discord. Younger friends offer fresh perspectives, while older ones impart hard-earned wisdom. "Plans fail for lack of counsel," Proverbs warns, "but with many advisers, they succeed" (Proverbs 15:22). Do your friendships span generations? Listening without judgment to different life experiences bridges divides and fosters mutual learning.

Also, travelling outside your comfort zone shakes up ingrained assumptions. As Mark Twain advised, "Travel is fatal to prejudice, bigotry, and narrow-mindedness." Exploring new places and cultures makes us more compassionate citizens of our world. Stepping outside the routine awakens creativity and problem-solving. Where might you venture out of familiar territory - physically, relationally, intellectually, spiritually - to encounter new views?

Then, recentering on God's awe combats cynicism. Regularly meditating on His majesty, from the vast cosmos to the intricacies of the human body, revives childlike wonder essential for learning. "Always be intoxicated in God," urged Saint Augustine. Awe transforms naturalism into transcendence and stimulates holy curiosity. Are you nurturing a sense of expectancy about what new facets of God you might encounter next?

Most importantly, pursuing an ever-deepening knowledge of Christ energizes lifelong learning. Paul counted everything as rubbish compared to "surpassing worth of knowing Christ Jesus my Lord" (Philippians 3:8). Just as the disciples walked three years with Jesus without exhausting His wonders, we can never plumb the depths of Christ in this lifetime. Eternity awaits more revelations of His glory! Does this beautiful truth increase your hunger to know Him more? Beloved, be wary of thinking yourself exempt from heeding wisdom or settling for spiritual complacency. God gifts us fellow sojourners - young and old - as teachers to spur a lifelong pursuit of Christ. With eternity ahead, why limit how God may sanctify and use you in the coming years? There are always new lessons to absorb, new revelations of Jesus' beauty. Stay hungry; stay humble. Joyful learning awaits at every turn. Our wise Teacher still has much to show those with a listening ear.

Conclusion

Beloved friends, we have explored the call to live with wholehearted devotion for the glory of Jesus Christ alone in the book **The Power of Relevant and Impactful Living,** which will become a reality via cultivating an intimate walk with Him through priority time in the Word, fervent prayer, and obedience to the Spirit's leading. Our great God deserves no less than our undivided love and abandonment of His purposes.

In a world full of distractions and lesser affections vying for our allegiance, we must fix our gaze upon the supremacy and beauty of Christ. He alone is worthy of our ceaseless adoration and longing. May the prayer of our hearts echo Paul's - to know Him in the power of His resurrection, sharing in His sufferings and becoming like Him in death, somehow attaining the resurrection from the dead (Philippians 3:10-11). Compared to the surpassing value of intimacy with Jesus, everything else fades to ash.

As the Master crafts and shapes us through the joys and trials of each season, let us respond with patience, trust in His wisdom, and gratitude for His redeeming love. In times of suffering, waiting, disappointment or uncertainty, repeatedly call to mind the Father's faithfulness on this journey. Not one promise has failed. He who began this good work in you will carry it to completion (Philippians 1:6). Rest confidently in that enduring truth.

No matter your age or station in life, God has assigned you to shine for Him right where you are planted. Bloom where you are planted. Bear magnificent Kingdom fruit through simple acts of devotion and service. What matters is not platform or achievements but humility, character, and faithfulness with what the Master entrusts to you. Finish each day knowing you have loved Him and others well.

Finally, brothers and sisters, let us keep our eyes fixed on Jesus, drawing strength from one another as we travel home to our eternal destiny. Though the trials we face today are but "light and momentary troubles", they are producing for us an eternal glory that outweighs them all (2 Corinthians 4:17). The day soon approaches when we will behold our Bridegroom face to face. Until then, live with joy and hope, beloved ones. Keep looking up - our redemption draws near! The Master is coming soon. May He find us faithful and fill us with the joy and hope of our eternal destiny.

My friends, you were created for such a time as this, to walk courageously as light in the darkness, hope to the hopeless, and salt that awakens spiritual thirst. Waste no time comparing yourself to others. Embrace the holy calling Christ has placed specifically on your life. You bear His image; you carry His Spirit. That makes you powerful beyond measure to touch this world for eternity. You have the power to make a significant impact. Go bravely into the adventures He has prepared for you! God is for you - who can stand against you? Abide in Him always. Our majestic Savior is worth it all.